COPD COMPASS

Therapies For Improved Lung Function And Quality Of Life

Navigate Chronic Obstructive Pulmonary Disease (COPD) With Therapies Aimed At Enhancing Lung Function And Respiratory Well-Being

DR. BRIDGET PROMISE

CHAPTER ONE

Introduction

The idea of weight management has evolved beyond conventional paradigms in the ever-changing field of health and wellness, giving birth to a holistic approach that acknowledges the connection between the mind and body.

This all-encompassing viewpoint recognizes that maintaining a healthy weight requires more than simply tracking calories or following a tight diet. In this investigation, we look into the holistic approach to weight health, comprehending the importance of physical exercise for balanced well-being, the critical function of nutrition, and the complex mind-body relationship.

Recognizing The Holistic Method For Weight Loss

The holistic approach to weight wellbeing focuses on a person's total health and happiness rather than just the outward look of their body.

It acknowledges that maintaining a healthy balance between the mind and body is just as important to weight control as just losing weight. This method takes into account several variables, such as stress management, lifestyle decisions, and emotional well-being, and it recognizes the critical roles these variables play in reaching and maintaining a healthy weight.

Adopting a holistic viewpoint entails realizing that problems related to weight are often complex. People struggle with their weight for a variety of reasons, such as psychological effects, environmental variables, and genetic predispositions. Recognizing the complexities of weight wellness allows people to approach their path with more compassion and understanding, emphasizing total health over giving in to social pressure or fast fixes.

Examining The Relationship Between Mind And Body In Weight Control

A key component of the holistic approach to weight health is the mind-body link. Our behaviors—including those about food and exercise—are greatly influenced by our ideas, feelings, and mental health.

For example, stress may lead to emotional eating, which can result in bad food choices and irregular eating habits. Long-term success in weight control requires an understanding of and attention to the underlying psychological problems that lead to weight difficulties.

A crucial element of the mind-body relationship is mindful eating. It entails developing a positive connection with food, being aware of hunger and fullness signals, and paying attention to the sensory experience of eating.

Eating mindfully may assist people in making thoughtful decisions, enjoying the tastes of food, and creating a healthy connection with food.

Furthermore, it's critical to address the emotional factors that lead to overeating or harmful behaviors. People who possess emotional intelligence and coping strategies may effectively manage stress, anxiety, and other emotional obstacles without turning to unhealthful eating habits. This all-encompassing strategy includes cultivating a mentality that promotes a healthy and long-lasting connection with food and body image in addition to behavior modification.

CHAPTER TWO

The Significance Of Diet In Maintaining A Sustainable Weight

A key component of the holistic approach to weight health is nutrition. Adopting a nutritious and well-balanced eating plan that satisfies individual nutritional demands is prioritized above fad diets or severe limitations.

Entire, high-nutrient meals serve as the cornerstone for long-term weight management by giving the body the vital vitamins, minerals, and macronutrients it requires for optimum performance.

With this method, people are encouraged to see food as nourishment for their bodies rather than a cause for shame or limitation. A well-rounded and fulfilling diet that supports an individual's overall health and weight objectives may be created by combining a range of fruits, vegetables, whole grains, lean meats, and healthy fats.

A more thoughtful and pleasurable meal experience is also enhanced by mindful eating techniques like watching portion amounts and eating slowly.

The holistic approach to nutrition is significant because it takes individual preferences and variances into account. It acknowledges that there isn't a single, universally applicable remedy and exhorts individuals to discover a dietary regimen that suits their requirements and way of life.

This adaptability helps maintain weight healthiness over time by improving adherence to a healthy eating plan and cultivating a pleasant connection with food.

Including Exercise For A Balanced Well-Being:

A key element of the holistic approach to weight health is physical exercise. Apart from its function in burning calories and aiding in weight reduction, consistent exercise enhances general health and wellness.

It supports the preservation of lean muscle mass and has a good effect on mood, energy levels, and cardiovascular health.

The holistic approach to physical exercise places a strong emphasis on the value of engaging in activities that people love. The idea is to partake in activities that make you happy and fulfilled, whether that means dancing, running, walking, swimming, or yoga. This improves the sustainability of exercise and fosters a favorable attitude toward physical activity.

It is also stressed that adding strength training to the exercise regimen is important since it helps to retain muscle mass, increase metabolism, and promote functional fitness. To enhance general health and fitness, the holistic approach recommends a well-rounded regimen of cardiovascular, strength, and flexibility training.

Additionally, exercise is acknowledged as a very effective stress-reduction strategy. Frequent exercise has been shown to lower stress hormones, lessen depressive and anxious symptoms, and enhance mental toughness in general. People may improve their capacity to handle life's obstacles by addressing the mind-body link via physical exercise, which helps to promote a more holistic and well-rounded approach to weight well-being.

In summary, the holistic approach to weight well-being highlights the connection between the mind and body and signifies a paradigm change in our knowledge of health.

People may control their weight in a more compassionate and long-lasting way by acknowledging the complexity of weight issues and taking care of the mind-body link. In this journey, nutrition is crucial since it promotes a healthy, well-balanced diet that supports general health.

Incorporating physical exercise also serves as a way to improve overall wellness by supporting resilience on the mental and emotional levels in addition to weight management. A good connection with one's body may be cultivated, leading to long-term health and happiness, by adopting a holistic approach to weight wellness.

Medication To Control Symptoms

Using drugs to treat infections, reduce inflammation, and ease airway tightness is a common strategy for managing COPD symptoms. Breathing becomes easier with the use of bronchodilators, which include long-acting beta-agonists (LABAs) and short-acting beta-agonists (SABAs). LABAs alone or in conjunction with inhaled corticosteroids may help lessen inflammation of the airways.

Anticholinergics are a different family of drugs that are often utilized in the treatment of COPD. These medications aid in clearing the airways and lowering mucus production. To give complete symptom relief, combination inhalers containing both corticosteroids and bronchodilators are used in certain patients.

Antibiotics for bacterial infections and oral steroids for inflammation management may be recommended for individuals experiencing exacerbations or acute respiratory infections.

The degree of symptoms, the patient's medical history, and the particulars of their COPD all play a role in the tailored medicine selection process.

CHAPTER THREE

Inhalation Treatments To Enhance Respiratory Performance

When it comes to managing COPD, inhalation treatments are essential since they provide medicine directly to the lungs, which results in quicker relief and fewer side effects than oral medication. Nebulizers, dry powder inhalers, and metered-dose inhalers (MDIs) are frequently used equipment for delivering these treatments.

A precise synchronization between inhalation and medication release is necessary for the pressurized delivery of a measured dose of medication through MDIs. DPIs are an excellent option for patients who may have difficulty with the coordination needed for MDIs because they administer powdered medication that is activated by the patient's breath. Patients with severe COPD frequently use nebulizers, which turn liquid medication into a fine mist for easier inhalation.

Because they directly target the respiratory system and reduce systemic adverse effects, inhalation treatments are the recommended method. The patient's capacity to operate the device and the particulars of their treatment plan will determine which inhalation device and medication is best for them.

Changes In Lifestyle For Patients With COPD

A key element of managing COPD is changing one's lifestyle; this involves minimizing exposure to aggravating factors and enhancing general health.

People with COPD must stop smoking because it aggravates symptoms and speeds up the course of the illness. To help people stop smoking, there are support groups and counseling services that deal with the mental and physical components of addiction.

It's important to stop smoking in addition to limiting your exposure to irritants and pollutants in the environment. When there is poor air quality, it is recommended that people with COPD stay indoors, use air purifiers, and take other steps to minimize indoor pollution. Reducing occupational exposure to respiratory irritants is also important, and in some circumstances, mask use or other protective measures may be advised.

An essential component of managing COPD is nutrition. It's critical to maintain a healthy weight because being overweight can put a strain on the respiratory system. Maintaining strength and energy levels is crucial for people with COPD, and this requires proper nutrition. To guarantee that patients receive the right nutrition while managing any comorbidities, dietary counseling may be advised.

Programs For Exercise And Rehabilitation

Regular exercise is a cornerstone of COPD management, contributing to improved respiratory function, increased stamina, and enhanced overall well-being. Exercise helps strengthen respiratory muscles, improves cardiovascular health, and increases endurance. Pulmonary rehabilitation programs, which combine exercise training, education, and psychological support, are designed to empower individuals with COPD to better manage their condition.

Pulmonary rehabilitation typically includes supervised exercise sessions tailored to the individual's fitness level and goals. Education sessions cover topics such as proper breathing techniques, energy conservation strategies, and medication management. Psychological support, often in the form of counseling or support groups, addresses the emotional challenges associated with living with a chronic respiratory condition.

Home exercise programs are also recommended for individuals who may not have access to formal pulmonary rehabilitation centers. Simple activities, such as walking, cycling, and stretching, can be adapted to individual abilities and preferences.

In conclusion, the treatment approaches for COPD encompass a multi-faceted strategy that combines medications, inhalation therapies, lifestyle modifications, and exercise programs. A personalized approach, considering the individual's symptoms, disease severity, and overall health, is crucial for effective COPD management. By addressing both the symptoms and underlying causes, individuals with COPD can lead more fulfilling lives, managing their condition and improving their overall quality of life.

CHAPTER FOUR

Nutritional Strategies For COPD Management

Proper nutrition plays a crucial role in managing COPD, as individuals with this condition often experience difficulties in maintaining a healthy weight and energy levels. A balanced diet can help enhance overall well-being and mitigate the impact of COPD symptoms.

Focus On Nutrient-Rich Foods

Incorporating nutrient-dense foods into the daily diet is vital for individuals with COPD. Fresh fruits, vegetables, lean proteins, and whole grains provide essential vitamins and minerals that support respiratory function. These foods also aid in maintaining muscle strength, which is often compromised in COPD patients.

Maintain Adequate Hydration

Adequate hydration is paramount for individuals with COPD. Staying well-hydrated helps in thinning mucus secretions, making it easier to clear the airways. This is especially effective during exacerbations of COPD symptoms.

Consideration Of Energy Expenditure

COPD can increase the energy expenditure of individuals due to the extra effort required for breathing. Therefore, it's crucial to tailor caloric intake to meet the specific needs of the patient. Consulting with a healthcare professional or a nutritionist can help determine an appropriate dietary plan.

Oxygen Therapy And Its Role

For individuals with advanced COPD, supplemental oxygen therapy is often a key component of the treatment plan. Oxygen therapy helps ensure that the body receives enough oxygen to function optimally, relieving symptoms and improving quality of life.

Understanding Oxygen Saturation Levels

Monitoring oxygen saturation levels is essential in determining the need for supplemental oxygen. Healthcare providers assess blood oxygen levels through pulse oximetry, and when levels drop below a certain threshold, supplemental oxygen may be prescribed to maintain adequate oxygenation.

CHAPTER FIVE

Types of Oxygen Delivery Systems

There are several oxygen delivery methods, each tailored to meet distinct demands. Continuous oxygen flow devices and portable oxygen concentrators give flexibility for persons to keep an active lifestyle while guaranteeing a steady oxygen supply.

Compliance And Lifestyle Integration

Compliance and lifestyle integration are necessary for oxygen therapy-assisted COPD management to be successful.

Patients must be aware of the significance of consistently taking oxygen as directed by their medical professionals. Including oxygen therapy in everyday routines may improve general health and performance.

Surgical Interventions For Severe Cases

In severe instances of COPD when conservative therapy may not be effective, surgical procedures become a concern. These operations attempt to enhance lung function and general quality of life for those in the late stages of the illness.

Lung Volume Reduction Surgery (Lvrs)

LVRS is a surgical treatment that includes removing diseased parts of the lung. By lowering the capacity of the lungs, the remaining tissue can operate more effectively. This technique is often explored for persons with emphysema.

Lung Transplantation

An alternative for some people with end-stage COPD may be a lung transplant. This entails using healthy donor lungs to replace one or both of the damaged lungs. Lung transplantation is a complicated process with possible hazards that have to be carefully considered, even if it may greatly enhance the quality of life.

Alternative and Complementary Medicine

Many people with COPD investigate complementary and alternative therapies in addition to traditional medical treatments to better manage their symptoms and enhance their general health.

Breathing Exercises And Yoga

People with COPD may benefit from yoga and particular breathing exercises because they strengthen their respiratory muscles and help them relax.

Breathing exercises that emphasize regulated breathing assist in the management of dyspnea and enhance lung capacity.

CHAPTER SIX

Traditional Chinese Medicine And Acupuncture

Some people use traditional Chinese medicine and acupuncture to alleviate the symptoms of their COPD. By attempting to restore the body's energy balance, these methods may help lower inflammation and enhance respiratory health.

Supplements With Herbs

Some herbal remedies, including turmeric and ginseng, are thought to have anti-inflammatory qualities and might help further with COPD symptoms. Before adding any supplements to the treatment plan, it is essential to speak with medical specialists.

Handling Flare-Ups Of COPD

Exacerbations, another name for COPD flare-ups, may be difficult and may need immediate medical attention to stop the condition from becoming worse. The stability of long-term COPD therapy depends on the effective control of flare-ups.

Early Symptom Identification

It is essential to inform people with COPD about the early warning indicators of exacerbations. Timely intervention is made possible by identifying signs such as reduced exercise tolerance, color changes in sputum, and increasing dyspnea.

Medication Adherence And Action Plans

Creating and following a customized action plan for COPD is essential to controlling flare-ups. Typically, this plan outlines how to take medication modifications, when to visit a doctor, and how to manage symptoms on your own.

Programs For Pulmonary Rehabilitation

By taking part in pulmonary rehabilitation programs, people with COPD may acquire the abilities and information necessary to properly handle flare-ups. These courses often involve emotional support, fitness routines, and breathing exercises.

In summary, treating COPD requires a thorough and customized strategy that takes into account several facets of the illness. A comprehensive strategy may greatly enhance the quality of life for those with COPD, ranging from dietary plans to surgical procedures and complementary treatments. Moreover, stability and halting additional respiratory deterioration depend on the efficient treatment of COPD flare-ups. To create a treatment plan that meets each patient's unique demands and takes into account the unique obstacles presented by COPD, always seek the advice of medical specialists.

COPD Patients' Access To Emotional And Psychological Support

It may be difficult to live with COPD since it affects not only one's physical health but also one's mental and emotional stability. The constraints placed upon them by the condition may cause worry, melancholy, or a feeling of loneliness in the patient. Hence, for COPD patients to manage the psychological and emotional toll that their illness has on them, emotional and psychological assistance is crucial.

1. Therapy and Counseling: Attending therapy or counseling sessions may be quite helpful for those with COPD. Mental health specialists may provide coping mechanisms and a secure environment for people to voice

concerns, assisting them in navigating the emotional difficulties brought on by long-term sickness.

2. Support Groups: Participating in COPD support groups fosters empathy and a feeling of belonging. Engaging with those experiencing comparable difficulties may alleviate emotions of loneliness and provide a forum for exchanging insights, advice, and consolation.

3. Education and Coping Mechanisms: Two of the most important aspects of emotional support are learning about COPD

and creating coping mechanisms. Patients might feel more empowered and have less worry if they understand the condition and adopt practical symptom management techniques.

4. Family and Caregiver Involvement: It is essential to include family members and caregivers in the process of providing emotional support. Within the family, open communication promotes understanding and a nurturing atmosphere.

CHAPTER SEVEN

COPD In Particular Groups

Different demographics are affected by COPD, and some populations—like the elderly or those in severe stages of the disease—need specialized treatment.

1. COPD patients in their senior years: Age-related issues may provide extra obstacles for the elderly. It's critical to address COPD's possible effects on mental health in addition to its physical manifestations. Comprehensive care for senior COPD patients includes social interaction, help

with everyday tasks, and routine check-ins.

2. Advanced Stage COPD: People with advanced COPD may need more comprehensive care. Palliative care and conversations around last wishes grow to be significant components of medical treatment. It's critical to provide patients and their families with emotional assistance during this trying time.

3. Programs for Pulmonary Rehabilitation: Targeted pulmonary rehabilitation services address the various requirements of individuals with COPD. These

programs often combine physical activity, instruction, and emotional support to meet the particular difficulties that certain communities experience.

Maintaining COPD At Home

The treatment of COPD is not only done in clinical settings; a large portion of care is given at home. For COPD patients, home care techniques increase their quality of life.

1. Oxygen Therapy at Home: It's important to make sure oxygen is used correctly at home since many COPD patients need extra oxygen. Patients and their caregivers feel

empowered when they are informed about emergency procedures, safety precautions, and equipment maintenance.

2. Medication Management: Taking prescription drugs as directed is essential to controlling the symptoms of COPD. Effective home care requires setting up a regimen for taking medications and monitoring doses.

3. Making Your House COPD-Friendly: It's important to adapt your house to the requirements of people with COPD. This might include clearing out any respiratory irritants, making sure

there is enough ventilation, and positioning furniture to reduce physical strain.

4. Family and Caregiver Education: Effective home care for people with COPD requires educating family members and caregivers on how to manage the disease. This includes spotting exacerbation symptoms, giving medicine, and providing emotional support.

Organizations And Resources That Are Helpful

Support for COPD sufferers and their families is provided by a plethora of organizations and services. These organizations are essential in terms of information sharing, facilitating connections between people who have similar experiences, and giving support in several ways.

1. American Lung Association: This organization provides a plethora of information about COPD, including advocacy tools, instructional materials, and support groups.

2. COPD Foundation: The COPD Foundation offers a variety of tools, including community support and instructional materials. Their programs are

designed to make life better for those who have COPD.

3. Better Breathers Clubs: These support groups, which are often connected to community centers or hospitals, provide a safe space for COPD sufferers to talk about their experiences and gain knowledge from one another.

4. The National Heart, Lung, and Blood Institute (NHLBI) offers tools, research updates, and in-depth information about COPD to medical professionals as well as patients.

Summary

A crucial part of managing COPD is providing patients with emotional and psychological care, which takes into account their mental and emotional health in addition to their physical symptoms. Care must be customized for certain groups, such as the elderly and people with severe illnesses.

A thorough training program for family members and caregivers, along with environmental adjustments, are all important components of home care for people with COPD. When it comes to giving people with COPD information, a sense of community, and support, supportive resources and organizations are essential. COPD patients may greatly enhance their overall quality of life by adopting a holistic strategy that includes medical treatment along with practical and emotional assistance.